EVERY ONE'S DIET

EVERY ONE'S DIET

DR. NADIAH MOUSSAWI

Library of Congress Control Number: 2019913343
ISBN: Hardcover   978-1-7960-5719-5
                   Softcover   978-1-7960-5718-8
                   eBook   978-1-7960-5717-1

Print information available on the last page.

Rev. date: 03/09/2020

To order additional copies of this book, contact:
Xlibris
1-888-795-4274
www.Xlibris.com
Orders@Xlibris.com
798798

Dr. Nadiah Moussawi

PT, Dtp, RD, MSc, PhD

It all started one day, when I was on a radio program. The two guys sitting with me (producer and interviewer) were overweight, with big bones. The producer talked to me.

> Him: You drink a lot of water. Look at me, I am never thirsty.
>
> Me: I am always thirsty, and if I am not, I drink water because I am stressed out, bored, thinking about something, or even to change my mind, my mood.

It's funny because usually when I do the bodymetrix machine or body composition analysis (it's a test to know the percentage of water, muscle, fat, bones in the body) at the clinic, I found that the heavier a person is, the less water percentage they have in their body. Also, the results of that test after weight-loss diet would give me a higher water percentage for the same person, and usually in people with ideal or healthy weight a higher percentage of water content.

It has always intrigued me! I know that 60–70 percent of our body is composed from water, a higher body-fat mass would contain less water, and a higher muscle mass would contain more water.

All of these facts lead me to answer the following questions:

1. Do overweight people have less water in their body?
2. Do fit people have more water in their body?
3. Is water percentage the cause or one of the causes of being overweight?
4. Why do I suggest that people drink water to lose weight?
5. Can we have a simple diet (that I will name the *Everyday's Diet*) using water to lose weight and maintain it?

In order to answer all of these questions in a scientific way and to conclude on a scientific diet using water, dear reader, accompany me in my analytical escape that I will do my best to make simple, initially for me and then for you.

If you're not interested in the **WHY** of the *Everyday's Diet*, then jump to the section on how to follow the *Everyday's Diet*.

Let me tell you that for years I worked with overweight and obese people, and the most difficult thing I find is dieting. Food is a need, a social activity, a stress release, an activity, a pleasure. The objective of this book is to show you that even if you should lose weight, afterward you should maintain it. This book discusses the importance of water in your everyday diet and how to include water and watery food in your meals, snacks, and lifestyle in order to lose weight and to maintain it for good (or at least a long time).

Dear reader, dieting is not something temporary. It is not an antibiotic that, after taking it for a time, you get rid of it like an infection! Diet is about the modification of your food habits and lifestyle in a way that it doesn't affect your life and/or well-being. So when you do the *Everyday's Diet*, you should continue with water-drinking habit, including the timing and quantity, as written for the rest of your life.

How much can you lose?

The *Everyday's Diet* is a medium approach to losing weight. I mean, no one is running after you to lose in three or seven or ten days!

Take a Breath!

The *Everyday's Diet* will take from four to eight weeks to reduce your weight or provide a visual result.

The *Special Everyday's Diet* will take from two to six weeks, and you will see the result.

What I say to my patients: "You are not a model, and anyway, being a model is for a certain age! The weight-loss program should be in a healthy way, respecting your body, needs, and social life; and the objective should be your health [knee pain, back pain, diabetes risk, hypertension risk, high cholesterol risk, cancer risk, problem of breathing when walking, sleeping, etc.] and then your image!"

I mean, you can work on your image with a designer or hairdresser or makeup artist, or simply by being inspired from some design magazines or websites! Beauty is subjective, and it is all about proportionality. Health is objective, and it is all about precise numbers (blood sugar, blood pressure, healthy weight, etc.), well-being, and your feelings.

Then let's focus on our health and well-being!

Following this diet, your body might react differently. It depends on your genes, metabolism rate (how many calories or how much energy you burn per hour), exercise level, how and when you eat, your gender, your daily sleep, and your stress level. So we are not equal— we have different and realistic backgrounds that we should respect, but with simple modifications, we would see a result at the end!

This book is a sweet combination of the theory I have learned, my experience, and my reflection throughout the years.

Let's see some scientific and proved facts.

Approximately 60–70 percent of the human body is made of water, both inside and outside the cells. Water is everywhere in your body (in your brain, muscles, bones, cells, etc.) so it plays a vital role. Water is primordial to life because it is the most abundant component in our blood. A human being cannot survive more than few days without water because we cannot reserve big quantities of water. Some animals beat us for the water reserve. For example, camels, ostriches, and giraffes (who beat camels).

Let us focus on the human body.

This is the distribution of the 60–70 percent water content in your body:

- Muscles, 75 percent
- Brain, 75 percent
- Bones, 22 percent
- Fat tissue, 10 percent

Muscles contain more water because of their composition that's higher in glycogen (glucose in the muscle). That sugar is used as fuel when you do exercises (physical activity), mostly. That means that athletes have more glycogen, so more water is in their body compared to sedentary (nonactive) people.

Gender Difference

If you are a man, you have approximately 60 percent of water in your body, because your muscle weight is greater. If you are a woman, you have approximatively 55 percent of water in your body, because you have more fatty tissues (around the breast and uterus), which is necessary for reproduction. That's true for two people from different gender with the same weight, same age, and same level of physical activity.

Age Differences

At birth, as a baby you had approximately 78–80 percent of water content, and at your first birthday, that percentage drops to 65 percent. The more you advance in age, the more you lose muscle weight and the less you have water in your body. Probably, that is the reason why they say you have slower metabolism (calorie-burning process) as you age! In fact, the elderly have approximately 50 percent of water in their body.

How Is Water Lost?

Generally, by

- Urination
- Bowel movement
- Breathing
- Perspiration (depends on your daily activity, health status, and the climate)

You lose water every minute through breath, sweat, and bowel movement.

Dehydration Causes

Pregnancy (Women)

- The plasma volume, roughly the body's blood, increases, especially at the last trimester (six to nine months). We know that plasma, or the blood, is mainly composed of water.
- Approximately 85 percent of the placenta volume is water.
- The fetus itself is composed of 70–90 percent water.
- The EFSA (European Food Safety Authority) recommends an increase of 300 ml of water per day for pregnant women.

Breastfeeding (Women)

- About 85–88 percent of human milk is made from water, so the need for water should be increased during lactation (breastfeeding).
- The EFSA recommends an increase of 700 ml of water per day for this category of women.

Exercise (Physical Activity)

When you do exercise and you sweat, you lose water in addition to some minerals, especially if you exercise during warm temperatures (indoor or outdoor). Drinking water would replace and restore your loss of water, would improve blood circulation, and would help your body to regulate your body temperature, and finally, would enhance your performance.[1]

According to a study published in 1995, in the *European Journal of Applied Physiology and Occupational Physiology*, replacing fluid (water with some minerals such as sodium, potassium, etc.) after exercising can be achieved by drinking water along with a snack that provides a significant amount of electrolytes, like sodium or potassium. A banana, for example, or a liquid enriched with minerals, like a sports drink.

It depends on the level of exercise and exercise type, but for athletes and/or sportive types (especially with high-intensity and/or high-endurance activities like jogging) is better to drink before, during, and after exercise. In addition to that, if you find out that you lost weight after your session of exercise, that means you are dehydrated; it is then important to replace the fluids you lost (500–750 ml, or 16–25 oz, for every pound, 0.5 kg, you lost). However, a cup of water, 250 ml (8 oz), for every thirty minutes of moderate exercise is recommended.

---

[1]   (E. D. Goulet, "Review," *Nut Rev*, 2012)

Medication Intake

Medicine like diuretics help release the body's water from the body via urination. Other medicine are phenothiazines and anticholinergics.

Diseases

These are like kidney diseases, diabetes, diarrhea, fever, or vomiting. Some infections or viruses (such as what causes urinary tract infection) are also in this group.

Food Intake

If you have noticed, when you eat a heavy meal that is rich in fat and/or in sugar and/or in salt and/or in spices and/or in fiber, you feel that your mouth is dry and you are thirsty. Why is that?

1. *Excessive sugar intake.* With a high sugar intake, your body tries to reserve the sugar excess (glycogen). For this process, it needs water. So you need more water!
2. *Excessive salt intake.* The body needs more salt to dilute the blood in order to return the level of sodium (salt) to normal and keep the balance. So you need more water!
3. *Excessive spice intake.* Spices increase slightly your body temperature (metabolism) so you might feel thirsty.
4. *Excessive fat intake.* Your body needs bile to digest fat in the liver. The composition of bile is 97 percent water. In addition to that, bile acids need water in the intestine to dissolve food fatty acids. After a fatty meal, you need more water!
5. *Excessive fiber intake.* Usually fiber need more water to be absorbed, so you might feel thirst.[2]

---

[2] (Myriam et al., "Re-evaluation of the Mechanisms of Dietary Fiber and Implications for Macronutrient Bioaccessibility, Digestion and Postprandial Metabolism," *Br J Nutr*, 2016)

6. *Some vegetable consumption like asparagus, parsley, celery, and artichokes.* These vegetables have diuretic properties (more urination), so you feel thirsty after having them.
7. *Excessive alcohol intake, caffeine-based beverages.* Alcohol and caffeine are diuretics, so you excrete more when you drink alcohol or caffeine-base beverages.
8. *Excessive protein intake, such as in the protein diet.* The body needs more water to metabolize nitrogen intake in protein food items such as meat or protein powder.

Being Stressed Out and Dehydration

Stress can cause dehydration (thirst), and the opposite is true: thirst can cause stress. It is a vicious circle. When you are stressed out, your heartbeat is faster (blood circulation), and you breathe more heavily (sweat), so you need more water, more fluids. Under stress, your cortisol level is higher as well.[3]

Let's Continue with this Cortisol Hormone

Cortisol (a hormone) plays many roles in the body. One of them is its effect on our body weight. In fact, higher cortisol levels are linked with higher appetite, higher cravings for sugar and salt, so more calorie intake. We crave food!

In addition to that, it reduces testosterone release, leading to a reduced muscle mass and, in turn, to a lower metabolism (less calories burned). So when cortisol levels are high, it causes weight gain.

---

[3] (Gina Shaw, "Water and Stress Reduction: Sipping Stress Away," Webmed, 2009; Abraham et al, "Cortisol, Obesity and the Metabolic Syndrome: a Cross-Sectional Study of Obese Subjects and Review of the Literature." *Obesity*, 2013; E. S. Epel et al, "Stress and Body Shape: Stress-Induced Cortisol Secretion is Consistently Greater Among Women with Central Fat. *Psychosom Med*, 2000; P. M. Oeeke. Chrousos, "Hypercortisolism and Obesity." Ann NY *Acad Sci*, 1995.)

After reading these causes, can I say water intake is somehow linked to body weight? Let's see the scientific literature and conclude at the end.

Weight and Water

Overweight

A study has been conducted from 2009 to 2012 by Tammy Chang et al., and they found that people with inadequate hydration had a higher body weight. If you like to read more about this research, please don't hesitate to check out the reference below.[4]

There is a big review that someone conducted on the subject on 4,963 retrieved records done in 2013. They took all of these studies and compared their results. They found out that there was an association between increased water consumption (intake) and weight loss and weight maintenance in individuals following a diet. In addition to that, in order to get these results, drinking water is a habit that should be practiced for long period of time. The few studies that have not found any result was mainly because the conduction was on a shorter time frame.[5]

Water and Metabolism (Calorie Utilization)

In a study in "The Journal of Clinical Endocrinology and Metabolism" from 2003, metabolic rate (energy or fuel utilization) increases by 30 percent after drinking two cups of water.

Let's see how water helps to regulate or manage your weight.

---

[4]   (Tammy Chang, "Inadequate Hydration, BMI, and Obesity Among US Adults: NHANES 2009–2012," ***MPH2***)

[5]   (Rebecca M. et al., "Association between Water Consumption and Body Weight Outcomes: A Systematic Review," *The American J of Clin Nutr*, 2013.)

If you have less water in the body, you have less muscle mass, and your metabolism is lower. When you are dehydrated, your metabolism slows down. This affects your ability to burn fat. In addition to that, your body mistakes your need of water (thirst) for food intake, which increases your calorie consumption. So you eat more, and you accumulate more fat.

Higher Calorie Consumption

On the other hand, when you don't drink enough water, your kidney is affected. That means it cannot purify your blood from toxins properly (filter). That influences your liver to stop metabolizing fat cells, and finally, it slows down once again your metabolism. The excess of fat would be accumulated as a weight gain. Simply, when the filter is affected, it presses the engine (liver) to slow down the energy consumption, and the energy (fat) would accumulate because it is not utilized.

Slower Metabolism

As we saw, today scientific community have accepted that increasing water intake helps you lose weight and maintain it.[6]

Drinking Water and Calories Burning

First of all, water is a calorie-free beverage. Second, researchers found that drinking water would increase calories you burn in twenty-four hours (resting energy expenditure, energy you burn by lying down without doing any activity). It has been reported that resting calorie expenditure increases by 24–30 percent within ten minutes of drinking water (500 ml, 16 oz), and that process lasts for sixty minutes.

---

[6] (Muckelbauer et al., "Association between Water Consumption and Body Weight Outcome: A Systematic Review," *Am J Clin Nutr*, 2013)

A study reported that increasing the consumption of water by 1 liter (32 oz) in twenty-four hours for 12 months without any modification in physical activity and/or food intake would decrease the weight by 2 kg (4.4 lb).[7]

That's true even for kids. In a study conducted in seventeen schools, they found out after placing water fountain and encouraging children to drink water, that the risk of obesity was reduced by 31 percent for 1 school year (days kids were at school). [8]

Water and Appetite

Also the scientific community have agreed on the fact that drinking water before each meal reduce the weights. A study reported that adults who took a glass of water before their meal would lose 2 kg (4.4 lb) over 12 weeks—that without making any other modification. The explanation behind that is that the water occupy a volume in your stomach, so you end up eating less at that meal, as mentioned before. Yes, dear reader, it affects in a good way your high appetite and your cravings. It is a Natural appetite suppressor.[9]

---

[7] (Boschmann et al., 'Water-induced thermogenesis,' *J Clin Endocrinol Metab* 2003; E. A. Dennis et al., "Water Consumption Increases Weight Loss during a Hypocaloric Diet Intervention in Middle-Aged and Older Adults," *Obesity*, 2010; J. D. Stookey et al., "Drinking Water is Associated with Weight Loss in Overweight Dieting Woman Independent of Diet and Activity," *Obesity*, 2008.)

[8] (R. Muckelbauer et al., "Promotion and Provision of Drinking Water in Schools for Overweight Prevention: Randomized, Controlled Cluster Trial," *Pediatrics* 2009.)

[9] (E. L. Van Walleghen et al. "Pre-meal Water Consumption Reduces Meal Energy Intake in Older but Not Younger Subjects," *Obesity*, 2007; Len Kravitz, "Water: The Science of Nature's Most Important Nutrient, University of New Mexico; P Kendall, "Drinking Water Quality and Health," Colorado States University, 2010).

Dr. Nadiah Moussawi

Water and Weight Maintenance

Drinking more water is associated with maintaining weight after a
weight loss program

Generally, you gain 1.45–1.50 kg every four years. Making a habit
to drink water would force you to drink less other beverages (like
sweet beverages) you eat and drink less calories and you increase
your resting expenditure in twenty-four hours. In fact, studies have
reported people who drink water have, on average, less calorie intake
in 24 hours by almost 9–10 percent (180–200 calories less intake).[10]

So adding 1 cup, 250 ml (8 oz), of water per day, you have more
chances to maintain your weight for a longer period of time.

Is it possible that you are thirsty and you believe you are hungry? Yes,
it is. Apparently we have the same area in the brain for hunger and
thirst, but scientists are not sure from this information. So you might
be thirsty, but you think you are hungry. The best way to resolve this
in order to limit your caloric intake is, whenever you feel hungry, you
take one glass of water then you wait for fifteen to twenty minutes.
If the stomach is still grumbling, that means you are hungry. If not,
you were simply thirsty![11]

---

[10]   (B. M. Popkin et al., "Water and Food Consumption Patterns of US Adults
from 1999 to 2001," *Obes Res*, 2005; M. C. Danielle et al., "Impact of Water
Intake on Energy Intake and Weight Status: A Systematic Review," *Nutr Rev*,
2010; A. Pan et al., "Changes in Water and Beverage Intake and Long-Term
Weight Changes: Results from Three Prospective Cohort Studies," *Int J Obes*,
2013.)

[11]   (Jennifer Rabin, "True Hunger and False Cravings," *Mother Earth Living:
Natural Home, Healthy Life*, 2004.)

Dehydration Signs

Degree of dehydration can be classified in light and severe stages. Personally, I find it very wide and general as signs related to dehydration, but that's all we have!

Light
thirst
dry or sticky mouth
dry, cool skin
not peeing too much
dark color of pee, more yellow to brownish
headache
muscle cramps (especially days you're doing physical activities)

Severe
not peeing or having brown pee
very dry skin (you can scratch it)
dizziness
rapid breathing
rapid heartbeat
sunken eyes
fatigue, weakness
irritability
sleepy
fainting

Babies and Kids
dry mouth and tongue
no tears
dry diapers at least for 3 hours
sunken eyes, cheeks, and soft spot on the top of the skull
sleepy
weak and irritability

Does dehydration cause hormone imbalance? Yes, my dear reader, and this imbalance might be related to weight gain. Some examples are the following:

- Less testosterone levels, which might be caused by a disease or dehydration.
- Having less water in the body or being dehydrated affect some hormones, such as testosterone (male hormone) or insulin (sugar hormone) production levels.
- Being dehydrated decreases testosterone levels and increases insulin, and these alterations both increase belly fat and fat accumulation, so leading to weight gain.[12]

Elevated levels of the hormone angiotensin II (AngII) might be the cause of some diseases or dehydration. Higher AngII levels are associated with many chronic diseases, such as obesity, diabetes, cancer, and cardiovascular disease. This leads to weight gain.

Also dehydration might affect serotonin and tryptophan (mood hormones) levels that in turn affect our mood. Some researchers reported that dehydration causes depression and might worsen anxiety. As I mentioned the brain is composed of 75 percent of water, it is no wonder why.[13]

Some researchers reported that some infections such as urinary tract infection might be related to dehydration.[14]

---

[12] (R. J. Mughan et al., *European Journal of Applied Physiology and Occupational Physiology*, 1995; Kendall Hopwood, "Review Your Life, The H2O Factor: Hydration Supports Weight Loss, 2009.)

[13] (E. Lawrence et al., "Mild Dehydration Affects Mood in Healthy Young Women," *The Jou of Nutr*, 2012; P. Nathalie et al., "Effects of Changes in Water Intake on Mood of High and Low Drinkers," Public Library of Sciences, 2014)

[14] (R. Beetz, "Mild Dehydration: A Risk Factor of Urinary Tract Infection?" *J Clin Nutr*, 2003)

So being dehydrated affects our weight, appetite, fat accumulation, mood, hormone levels, and well-being!

Dangers of Dehydration

As we saw, dehydration can cause many complications. It might have a light sign, such as thirst, but it can lead to the more severe result, which is death. Fluid losses of 1 percent can lead to an elevation of your body temperature. If you lose between 3 and 5 percent of your body weight in fluid, it can affect the cardiovascular system (heart and arteries), and if you lose up to 7 percent of your body weight in fluid, you will collapse!

Can I Not Feel the Thirst?

There is a condition adipsia that is characterized by the absence of thirst, which is caused by a lesion in a specific area in the hypothalamus (brain). However, is a rare disease.

Some healthy people don't feel the thirst, is it possible they have lost the feeling? Logically, if water is vital to our body, then being thirsty is instinctive. How come some of my patients say they don't feel thirsty or they don't like to drink water?

I have not found a scientific answer but have some logical theories.

1. Water is vital for the body. People might take some other beverages, such as juices or something else, OR some food that contains a percentage of water (fruits and vegetables, soup or something else). These might compensate for the water need.
2. The body possess an ability of adaptation. Deprived of water, it switches to survivor mode. Given less water, it would ask for less.

3. Sometimes we are too busy or stressed out. We forget to drink, even if we are thirsty, and with time, we might lose the thirst sensation.
4. We don't like water because when drinking, we might develop acidity or a sensation of fullness or feel sickness of any sort. We associate water with sickness consciously or unconsciously.

There was a research (Tim Newman, "How Do Our Brains Tell Us We Are Thirsty?" *Medical News Today*, 2018) which examined the different components in the brain in relation to the thirst sensation. It is an amazing and complicated process, and it needs more research for some people who lost or don't feel thirst. My questions: Are there any degrees of thirst? How do we measure it scientifically? Can it be related to our instinctive feeling of thirst or to our percentage of fat?

Can I Be Drinking Too Much Water? And Is It Dangerous?

Yes, ladies and gentlemen, it might be dangerous! Like everything in life, the excess of water intake might harm you. As for water consumption excess, it is very rare, but it can happen. It was reported in athletes doing endurance exercises (for long periods). The body could not take the excessive quantity of water, so they would suffer from hyponatremia (dilution of sodium levels in the blood, less sodium in the body). It has been seen in soldiers as well. If hyponatremia continues, it would lead to death. Don't worry, it has not been seen in general public, only in athletes or soldiers. The concept behind that is this: the blood sodium levels would dilute with the water excess and would cause hyponatremia (less sodium in the body), which might cause body intoxication. According to scientific data, this intoxication is the result of drinking more than 5 gallons (18-19 l) of water in a period of a few hours. Current guidelines are 1–1.5 l

(32-50 oz) per hour during time of heavy sweating (athlete or soldier or people working outdoor for long hours).[15]

What I learned is that apparently, kidneys regulate the excess volume. In case of water excess, we know that kidneys can eliminate 20–28 l of water per day (5.3–7.4 gal) but it's hard for them to excrete more than 0.8–1 l of water per hour (28-32 oz). So you cannot decide to drink 3 l in one hour. You should distribute that quantity over twenty-four hours.[16]

What is the exact quantity to drink water?

We know water is vital to our body, but we don't know the exact quantity. According to experts, you should go with the color of your urine. Be careful because sometimes you might be hydrated, but some food intake like asparagus or carrot or beetroot might affect the urine color. Some other experts say when you are thirsty, be careful. Some scientific reports say that being thirsty is already a sign of dehydration. And according to my experience, some people don't feel the thirst![17]

We know that some factors affect water intake, such as exercise, working outdoors in a hot climate, diseases like type 2 diabetes, medicine, breastfeeding, etc.

---

[15] J. W. Gardner, "Death by Water Intoxication," *Mil Med*, 2002.
D. B. Speedy et al, "Exercise Associated Hyponatremia: A Review," *Emerg Med*, 2001.
MayoClinic.com, "Water: How Much Should You Drink Every Day?" April 2010.
Allison Aubrey, "Five Myths About Drinking Water," NPR.org, April 2008.
Coco Ballantyne, "Strange but True: Drinking Too Much Water Can Kill," ScientificAmerican.com, June 2007.

[16] (Min A Joo et al, "Hyponatremia Caused by Excessive Intake of Water as a Form of Child Abuse," *Annal of Ped Endo and Metab*, 2013.)

[17] (James McIntosh, "Only Drink When Thirsty to Avoid Health Risks," *Medical News Today*, 2015)

Dr. Nadiah Moussawi

What to do?

Let's make it simple: according to the Institute of Medicine,

- drink 9 cups (2 l) if you are a woman, and
- drink 12 cups (2.8 l) if you are a man.

From all beverages and food (some food are rich in water such as fruits and veggies), as total water intake (food, water, and beverages)

- 2.7 l, 91 oz, of total water as for woman, and
- 3.7 l, 125 oz, of total water as for man.

About 80 percent of water intake in North America comes from water and beverages, and the rest, 20 percent comes from food.[18]

However, body weight—which includes muscle mass, bone mass, fat mass, brain, blood, etc.—should be taken in consideration as for the quantity of water intake every day. That means a thin person does need less water compared to a heavier person. But water is not the only liquid. There's food and other beverages rich in water.

Food and Beverages That Are a Source of Water

Reference: Dietitians of Canada

Fluids to Choose From	**Tips**
Water	• Water is calorie-free and a great way to quench your thirst. • Add a slice of lemon or lime to make it more refreshing.

---

[18] (James McIntosh, "Only Drink When Thirsty to Avoid Health Risks," *Medical News Today*, 2015)

	• Drink tap water. You don't need to drink bottled water. • If you drink well water, it should be tested regularly.
Fruit or Vegetable Juice	• Limit your intake of fruit juices since they are high in calories and low in fiber. • Eat the fruit instead. • 125 ml (½ cup) of juice is a serving of fruits and vegetables. Make sure you choose 100 percent real fruit juice. • Avoid fruit drinks, cocktails, punches, or beverages, as they have sugar added and less nutrients.
Milk/Fortified Soy or Rice Beverages	• Aim for 500 ml (2 cups) of low-fat milk or alternatives (less than 2 percent MF) as part of your fluid intake for the day.
Soft Drinks	• Choose soft drinks less often. Regular soft drinks are high in calories and sugar and low in nutrients. Some soft drinks, such as colas, may also contain caffeine. • Diet soft drinks are calorie- and sugar-free but may still have caffeine.

Broth and Soups	<ul><li>Broth and broth-based soups can be a good source of fluid. However, most canned or dehydrated broths or soups are high in sodium (salt).</li><li>Try making your own or choose prepared broths or soups lower in sodium.</li></ul>
Sports Drinks	<ul><li>Sport drinks are usually not needed to keep hydrated when you exercise.</li><li>Water and a healthy diet will replace water and minerals lost during exercise. If you exercise very hard, in extreme weather, for a long time, or wear a lot of sports equipment, you may benefit from a sports drink.</li><li>For more information on sports hydration, see the additional resources below.</li></ul>
Tea and Coffee (e.g. herbal tea, regular and decaffeinated coffee/tea)	<ul><li>Coffees and teas are not dehydrating. Limit caffeine intake to about 400 mg per day. That is equal to 750 ml (3 cups) of black coffee or 1 l (4 cups) of black tea per day.</li><li>Drink herbal teas or decaf coffee if you want to have more than the recommended amount of caffeinated beverages.</li></ul>

	<ul><li>Limit specialty coffees and teas. They can be high in sugar.</li><li>If you are pregnant, limit your caffeine intake to 500 ml (2 cups) of coffee or 750 ml (3 cups) of tea.</li></ul>

Do people become overweight because they don't drink enough water and when it starts?

Few researches in the field have not found any association between water consumption and weight loss. However, it depends on the quantity of water, the sample's size, and their weight, and also timing of water intake during the day. All of these are variables that might affect the result, and in this book, I am not writing a review on the subject and neither questioning their statistical tests, so I won't criticize those articles. Although most of the scientific studies in the field have found that increasing water intake with or without any modifications in lifestyle help to lose weight in overweight and obese subjects.

My conclusion is YES, we might drink less than our needs, especially some days or weeks, because of hormonal imbalance, a temporary or chronic diseases, work (outdoor), level of exercise, type of food intake, level of stress, etc., as mentioned below. All of these factors are associated with our body's water becoming less, lower metabolism, less muscle mass, a high fat percentage, and with time, an increase in our weight. So water intake affects body weight directly or indirectly! Water can't be the only reason, but certainly it is one of the main reasons.

The Everyday's Diet

You should respect the time and the quantity. You can have cold or warm water. You can add some mint or basil leaves or a few cucumber or fruit slices in your water. Drinking cold water slightly increases the metabolism (because it will burn a few more calories), but please don't drink cold water when you wake up, and if you don't like cold water, don't force yourself.

Start the day with 1–2 glasses of water depending on your weight. If you are

- overweight: 1 glass (250 ml)
- obese: 2 glasses (500 ml)

Before breakfast 15–30 minutes: second glass of water (250 ml)

After breakfast 2–3 hours: third glass of water (250 ml)

Before lunch 15–30 minutes: fourth glass of water (250 ml)

After lunch 2–3 hours: fifth glass of water (250 ml)

Before dinner 15–30minutes: sixth glass of water (250 ml)

Before going to bed: seventh glass of water (250 ml)

One to two snacks a day (before the snack 10–20 minutes): eighth glass of water (250 ml)

If you eat only twice or thrice per day, then you should drink more between meals!

In order to increase the quantity of water in your twenty-four hours, do the following:

- You should include for every meal and for every snack at least one food item rich in water (from the chart)
- You should sweat! At least for ten minutes (three to four times per week)

- If you take food items from below, you should increase your water intake by one to two glasses of water
  o Caffeine: tea, coffee, chocolate, soft drink, or any drink with caffeine
  o Alcohol
  o Diuretics (medicine or herbal pills or laxatives)
  o Some vegetables such as celery or asparagus
  o Sweet or sugary food or beverages
  o Salty food or beverages or snack
  o Fatty food (deep fried, pastries, fried food)
  o Protein (animal sources or from powder)
- If you do exercise or you are depressed or you live in high altitude area
- If you breastfeed or you are pregnant, you shouldn't lose weight, you can drink water and the best is to be followed by a registered dietitian.

Why do I call it *'the Everyday's Diet?'*

- Because there is little effort to following it.
- Not that much of deprivation.
- Even the avoid list can be consumed with moderation.
- It is a healthy diet (hypocaloric), and it contains all food groups.
- These changes should be maintained after weight loss.
- You can find easily all the ingredients and at low price.
- And it works...you lose weight gradually and in a healthy way!

Now, let's *apply the Everyday's Diet.*

Menu

<u>*Day 1*</u>

You open your eyes, wake up: *1 glass of water*

Before breakfast 15–30 minutes: *1 glass of water*

Breakfast: 1 whole wheat bagel with 2 tablespoons of cream cheese or 30 g of cheese with lettuce or cucumber + 1 kiwi or ½ cup of berries

After 2 hours: *1 glass of water*

After 30 minutes, snack: 1 fruit or 1 fruit salad (½–1 cup) + 10–15 plain almonds

After 2 hours: *1 glass of water*

After 30–60 minutes, lunch: 1–3 cups of veggie soup (like minestrone, no cream) you can use 1–2 tablespoons of sour cream in your soup, with ½–1 cup of cooked beans (lentils, red, or white beans) with ½ cup of corn or pasta cooked in the soup, some spices like pepper, chili, cumin.

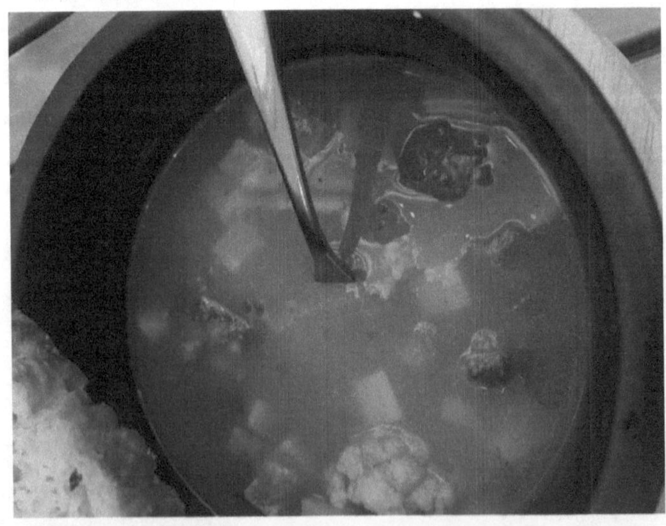

After 2 hours: *1–2 glasses of water*

Snack: 1 ice cream, light (100–120 calories), or 1 vanilla or chocolate pudding

Before dinner 30–60 minutes: *1 glass of water*

Dinner: grilled seafood—shrimp, scallops, or something else, 120–180 g, with garlic and lemon and butter with 4–10 tablespoons of cooked rice

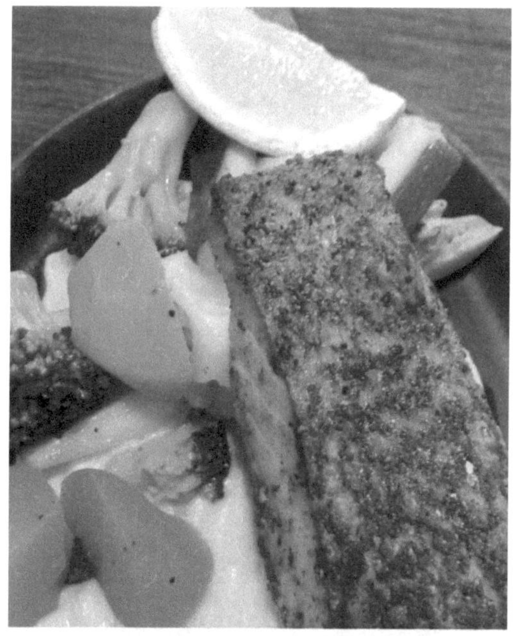

<u>Day 2</u>

You open your eyes, wake up: *1 glass of water*

Before breakfast 15–30 minutes: *1 glass of water*

Breakfast: 1 small muffin (oat or whole wheat or seeds) + 1 fruit + 1 plain yogurt

Dr. Nadiah Moussawi

After 2 hours: *1 glass of water*

After 30 minutes, snack: 2 cucumbers and 1 orange with 2–3 plain walnuts

After 2 hours: *1 glass of water*

After 30–60 minutes, lunch: tuna salad with balsamic vinegar and extra-virgin olive oil or nuts or avocado oil (tuna in water, 120–180 g, 2–3 cups of lettuce, 1 shredded carrot, chopped celery, fine herbs, salt and pepper)

After 2 hours: *1–2 glasses of water*

Snack: 1 small bag of chips baked in oven or 2 cups of popcorn

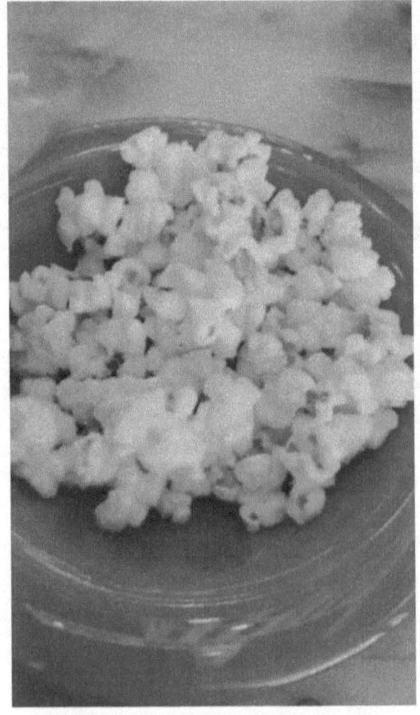

Before dinner, 30–60 minutes: *1 glass of water*

Dinner: chicken taoouk or grilled chicken with 3–4 tablespoons of hummus and 1 cup of tabolee with lettuce Or a salad with little of quinoa

<u>Day 3</u>

You open your eyes, wake up: *1 glass of water*

Before breakfast 15–30 minutes: *1 glass of water*

Breakfast: 1–2 pieces brown toast with 1–2 fried eggs, with or without 30 g of low-fat cheese and veggies (mushrooms, spinach, parsley)

After 2 hours: *1 glass of water*

After 30 minutes, snack: 5–10 baby carrots, cucumber, colorful pepper with 1 yogurt

After 2 hours: *1 glass of water*

After 30–60 minutes, lunch: 1–2 cups of lentil soup + 1–2 cups green salad (lettuce, cucumber, balsamic vinegar, and extra-virgin olive oil) + 1 smoothie (spinach leaves, ½ cup of Greek yogurt, ½ cup of 100 percent apple juice, ½ cup of carrot juice, ice cubes)

After 2 hours: *1–2 glasses of water*

Snack: 2 tablespoons of seeds or pistachio with 1 fruit

Before dinner 30–60 minutes: *1 glass of water*

Dinner: grilled fish or pan-fried fish, 120–180 g + 2 cups of grilled vegetables (zucchini, green beans, mushroom, broccoli) with fine herbs and lemon

Dr. Nadiah Moussawi

<u>Day 4</u>

You open your eyes, wake up: *1 glass of water*

Before breakfast 15–30 minutes: *1 glass of water*

Breakfast: $^1/_2$–$^3/_4$ cup of oats + 1 cup of low-fat milk + ½ cup of berries or 1 fruit or 1 small banana with cinnamon

After 2 hours: *1 glass of water*

After 30 minutes, snack: 1 kefir or 30 g of low-fat cheese, 2 crackers, 4–5 green olives

After 2 hours: *1 glass of water*

After 30–60 minutes, lunch: ½ cup of cooked couscous, 1–2 chopped chicory, 30–60 g mozzarella cheese, ½ cup of chopped parsley, 1 chopped tomato, 5–7 green chopped olive, 1–2 boiled and chopped beetroot, pepper, lemon, extra-virgin olive oil, cumin

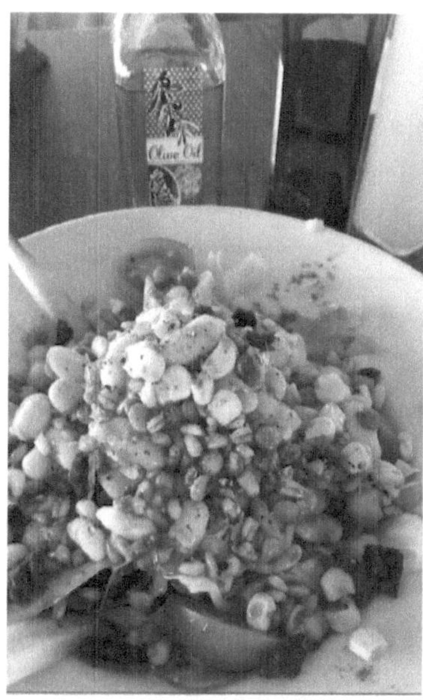

After 2 hours: *1–2 glasses of water*

Snack: 2 pieces of dark chocolate, 2 walnut

Before dinner, 30–60 minutes: *1 glass of water*

After 30–60 minutes, dinner: grilled chicken, 120–180 g, with lemon and fine herbs, with veggies (1 boiled potato, 1 cup of mushroom, ½ cup parsley, 1 tomato) dressing mayonnaise/mustard/lemon and fine herbs

Day 5

You open your eyes, wake up: *1 glass of water*

Before breakfast 15–30 minutes: *1 glass of water*

Breakfast: 1 brown English muffin with 1–2 poached eggs with ½ avocado with spinach (might be raw or cooked)

After 2 hours: *1 glass of water*

After 30 minutes, snack: 1 cup juice, 100 percent natural, 250–330 ml + 15–25 plain pistachios or peanuts (not salty, not sweet, not cheese-flavored, no spices)

After 2 hours: *1 glass of water*

After 30–60 minutes, Lunch: few pieces of sushi (4 pieces, and sashimi 3-5 pieces) with 1 cup of edamame

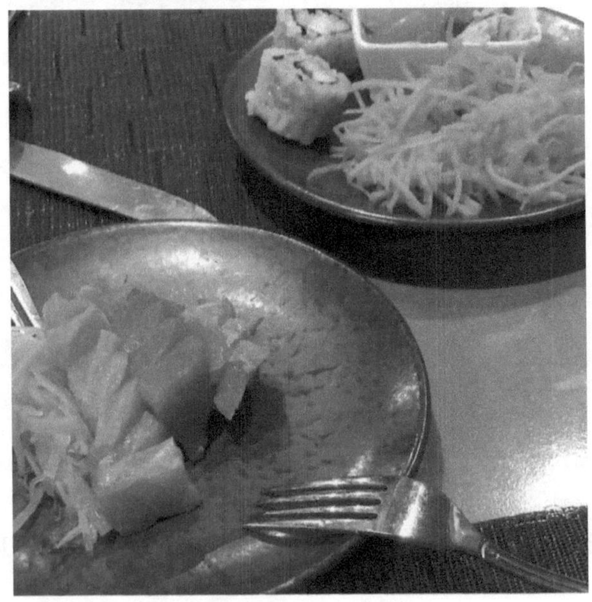

After 2 hours: *1 glass of water*

After 30 minutes, snack: 1 piece of dark chocolate (15 g) with 1 fruit

Before dinner 30–60 minutes: *1 glass of water*

Dinner: 1 cup of pineapple or berries with 1/2 cup of cottage cheese or 1/2 cup of Greek yogurt, 2 crackers whole wheat organic

<u>Day 6</u>

You open your eyes, wake up: *1 glass of water*

Before breakfast 15–30 minutes: *1 glass of water*

Breakfast: 1 cup fruit salad + ¾ cup cottage cheese or ½ cup ricotta cheese + 1–2 tablespoons plain seeds (not salty, not sweet, not spicy) and 1 teaspoon of chia seeds

After 2 hours: *1 glass of water*

After 30 minutes, snack: 1 granola bar or pudding (100 calories, no preservative agents) + 1 cup of low-fat milk

After 2 hours: *1 glass of water*

After 30 to 60 minutes, lunch: quinoa salad: 3–6 tablespoons of cooked bulgur or quinoa, 1 chopped tomato, 2–3 cups chopped of spinach or arugula, 2 tablespoons of pin seeds, ½–1 cup of broccoli or zucchini cooked and chopped, spices, balsamic vinegar and extra-virgin olive oil, fine herbs

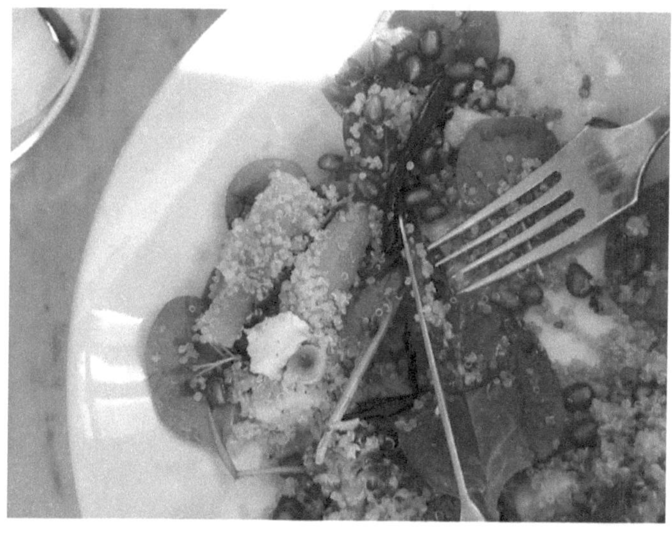

After 2 hours: *1–2 glasses of water*

Snack: 1 cup of fruit salad or 1 cup of mashed fruit (purée)

Before dinner 30–60 minutes: 1 glass of water

Dinner: ragout of veggies (onion, tomato, zucchini, eggplant, parsley, fine herbs) cooked with 5–7 meatballs or meat (lean minced meat with spices)

Day 6

You open your eyes, wake up: *1 glass of water*

Before breakfast 15–30 minutes: *1 glass of water*

Breakfast: ½ cup of beans cooked with ¾ of veggies (green pepper, tomato, onion, parsley, spices) with 1 egg with 1 sausage or 1 slice of turkey (lettuce and mustard)

After 2 hours: *1 glass of water*

After 30 minutes, snack: 1 cup of low-fat milk with 1 tablespoon of dried raisin or 2 dates or 1 dried fig

After 2 hours: *1 glass of water*

After 30 to 60 minutes, lunch: tuna sandwich (2 pieces brown toast or ½ brown baguette, 120–180 g tuna, 1–2 tablespoons of mayonnaise, pepper, fine herbs, chives, green pepper)

After 2 hours: *1–2 glass of water*

Snack: 1–3 pieces of dark chocolate, more than 55 percent of cacao, with 1 mandarin

Before dinner 30–60 minutes: *1 glass of water*

Dinner: grilled lean steak, 120–160 g, with 2 cup of vegetables (sautéed), mushrooms, leek, onion, bean sprouts, with soya sauce or fish sauce with sesame seeds

- Drink 1–2 glass of water before bed.
- As for dairy products or mayonnaise, you can choose low fat.
- As for the dark chocolate, 60 percent of cacao and more is considered dark. It is acceptable if you take the 50 percent of cacao, and progressively you increase the cacao content.
- It is a healthy diet, I would say hypocaloric one (less calorie). If you follow this diet for five days out of seven, with the water content as written, you will lose weight progressively.
- It is important that you do your best to sweat at least for ten minutes per day, at least for four days per week so you will drink more water, 1–2 cups depending on the intensity.
- Physical activity of any sort (exercises, simple fast walking, dancing, gripping the stairs, cleaning the house, gardening, playing with kids, having sex). Go according to your body and fitness intensity.
- For every coffee or caffeine drink you take, you should take the same equal quantity of water.
- For every 100 g of alcohol you take, you should drink 200 g of water. Limit your alcohol intake; it can increase weight.
- Try to have food and drinks that are enhanced with natural sugar, have no salt, are not fried, have no preservatives, are not spicy. Try to enhance the flavor of food with fine herbs, lemon, spices like cinnamon, saffron, cardamom, etc. If it happens that you take a salty, sweet, or oily high-protein snack or meal, you should drink more water, but only after 1–2 hours.
- Don't drink water or anything with your meal or snack— always before or after, as mentioned.
- You should drink more water if you are stressed out.

- Try to have always at least one item rich in water content at your snack or meal.
- As for the quantities in veggies or proteins, the minimum range mentioned is for people who are smaller (small frame of bones and weight) and the maximum range in the interval is for people who have bigger bones' frame.
- I will include some recipes rich in water so you can make them.
- Try always to choose food items that, when you read the ingredients list, is the shorter, and you get what is written. Make it simple: short list and comprehensible list with known words, no chemical or artificial flavors or preservation agents.
- Avoid the three white powders: sugar, salt, and white flavor (*avoid* means only have them 3–4 times per month) with moderation. Choose more whole wheat food rich in oats, seeds, or grains. Enhance the food flavors with fine herbs, lemon, ginger, and spices.
- You can have Mexican/Italian/Chinese dishes with rice or pasta and sauces, once per week.

If some of you want to lose weight faster, you can follow the *Special Everday's diet.* You can start with the *Everyday's Diet* and continue with the *Special Everyday's Diet.* If you suffer from a disease such as diabetes, hypertension, kidney problems, etc., it's better to discuss your diet with a health-care provider, and the best professional for that is a dietitian or nutritionist when it is related to food and nutrition.

How to apply *Special Everyday's Diet?*

When you open your eyes, you wake up: *1–2 glasses of water*

Before breakfast 30 minutes: *1–2 glasses of water*

Breakfast: 1 smoothie: in the blender, add ½ cup carrot juice, 1–2 tablespoons of iso protein, 1 tablespoon oat, ½ cup apple juice, ice cubes

After 2 hours: *1 glass of water*

After 30 minutes, snack: 1 fruit Or 1 fruit salad (1 cup) + 10–15 plain almonds

After 2 hours: *1 glass of water*

After 30 to 60 minutes, lunch: 2 cups of minestrone soup (veggies: zucchini, tomato, celery, potato, with red beans ½–1 cup) + 2 cups of green salad (lettuce, cucumber, green pepper) all dressed up with lemon and extra virgin olive oil.

After 2 hours: *1–2 glasses of water*

Snack: 2 tablespoon of seeds with 1 fruit

Before dinner 30–60 minutes: *1 glass of water*

Dinner: grilled fish or pan-fried fish, 120–180 g, + 2 cups of vegetables grilled (eggplant, mushroom, zucchini, broccoli) with fine herbs and lemon

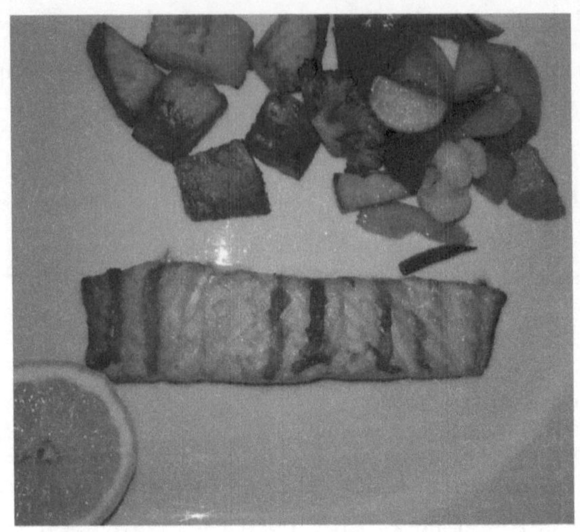

<u>Day 2</u>

When you open your eyes, you wake up: *1–2 glasses of water*

Before breakfast 30 minutes: *1–2 glasses of water*

Breakfast: 1 yogurt, ¾ cup berries (fresh or frozen), 2 tablespoons an high fiber cereal 1 teaspoon chia seeds, 1 teaspoon flax seeds, stevia

After 2 hours: *1 glass of water*

After 30 minutes, snack: 2 walnuts, 1 tablespoon of dried raisins, or 2 dates

After 2 hours: *1 glass of water*

After 30 to 60 minutes, lunch: 1 boiled potato + sauce: ½ cup red beans, ¼ cup chopped parsley or chives, 2–4 tablespoons of sour cream, pepper, 1 tablespoon chopped pickles or marinated tomato, 1 green or yellow chopped pepper

Before dinner 30–60 minutes: *1 glass of water*

Dinner: cabbage soup: 1 chopped onion, 2 cloves garlic, 2 cups chopped cabbage, ¼ cup chopped parsley, ¼ cup chopped coriander, 1 cup mushroom, 1 chopped carrot, 5–9 pieces shrimp, 1–2 tablespoons of oat, lemon, cumin, paprika, salt, pepper

In a pan, stir-fry the onion, garlic, parsley, and coriander for 3–5 minutes (medium heat) in 1 tablespoon of vegetable oil. Add the rest of ingredients, and add 2 cups of water and 1 cup of chicken or vegetable broth. Cover and cook for 15–20 minutes.

Add the spices and simmer for another 3–4 minutes and serve.

<u>Day 3</u>

When you open your eyes, you wake up: *1–2 glasses of water*

Before breakfast 30 minutes: *1–2 glasses of water*

Breakfast: in the blender, put ½ cup of orange juice, 1 boiled egg white, ¼ teaspoon vanilla extract, 2 tablespoons of lemon, 1 teaspoon of chia seeds, 1 teaspoon of whole wheat oats, ice cubes

After 2 hours: *1 glass of water*

After 30 minutes, snack: 1 yogurt or 1 kefir with 2 cucumbers and 1 orange

After 2 hours: *1 glass of water*

After 30 to 60 minutes, lunch: 1–2 cups of lentil soup + 2 cups of arugula salad with 1–3 tablespoon of plain sunflower seeds with balsamic vinegar and extra-virgin olive oil

After 2 hours: *1–2 glasses of water*

Snack: 1 ice cream, 120–150 calories, or 1 fruit yogurt

Before dinner, 30–60 minutes: *1 glass of water*

Dinner: 1 cup of edamame with chili sauce + 1–2 cups of tzatziki (1 cup of yogurt, 2 diced cucumbers, ¼ cup chopped mint, salt and pepper; you can add ½ brown pita grilled)

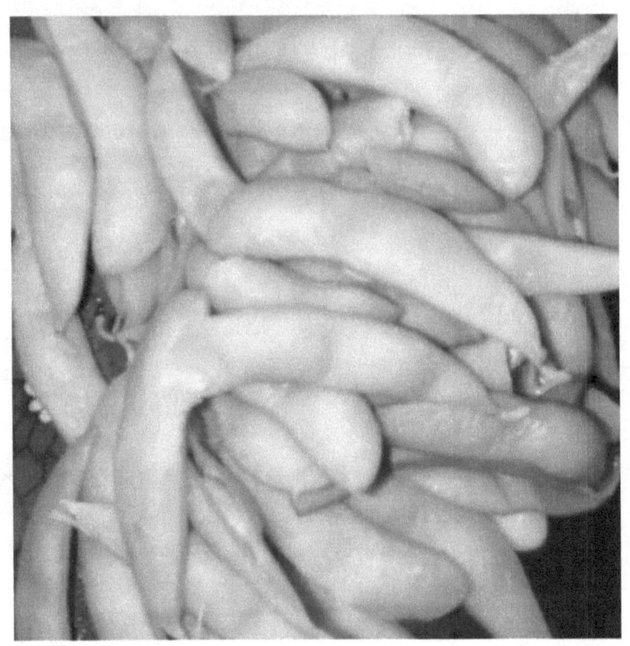

Day 4

When you open your eyes, you wake up: *1–2 glasses of water*

Before breakfast 30 minutes: *1–2 glasses of water*

Breakfast: $^1/_2$–$^3/_4$ cup whole wheat oats, 1 cup of low-fat milk, cinnamon, nutmeg, 1 banana, 1 teaspoon of chia or flax seeds

After 2 hours: *1 glass of water*

After 30 minutes, snack: 1 cup of veggies (tomato, pepper, mushrooms, celery) + 30 g of low-fat cheese

After 2 hours: *1 glass of water*

After 30 to 60 minutes, lunch: 1 cup of Greek yogurt with chives and lemon + 1–2 cups of boiled veggies (broccoli, carrot, cauliflower, green beans) with lemon

After 2 hours: *1–2 glasses of water*

Snack: 2–4 pieces of dark chocolate with 55 percent or more of cacao, with 1–2 kiwi fruits

Before dinner 30–60 minutes: *1 glass of water*

Dinner: 1–2 cups ragout of veggies (onion, eggplant, zucchini, tomato, pepper and salt) + ½–1 cup of cooked chickpeas

Day 5

When you open your eyes, you wake up: *1–2 glasses of water*

Before breakfast 30 minutes: *1–2 glasses of water*

Breakfast: in the blender: 1 cup of low-fat milk, ½–1 cup of papaya, stevia, 1-2 tablespoons of iso protein powder vanilla or your favorite flavor, 1 teaspoon of flax seeds

After 2 hours: *1 glass of water*

After 30 minutes, snack: 1 vanilla or dark chocolate pudding

After 2 hours: *1 glass of water*

After 30 to 60 minutes, lunch: grilled salmon 120–180 g + 2 cups of boiled or grilled vegetables (zucchini, broccoli, carrot, cauliflower)

After 2 hours: *1–2 glasses of water*

Snack: 2 tablespoon of seeds with 1 fruit

Before dinner 30–60 minutes: *1 glass of water*

Dinner: beetroot salad: 1–2 chopped boiled beetroot, ½ cup of chopped parsley, 2 cups of spinach, 30–60 g of goat cheese, olive oil and balsamic vinegar or lemon + 1 small piece of bread (whole wheat)

1–2 glasses of water before bed

Let's have some recipes that are for breakfast.

Oat and blueberries
$^1/_2$–$^3/_4$ whole wheat oats
½ blueberries or 1 unpeeled and chopped apple
3–5 tablespoons of Greek yogurt
cinnamon and chia seeds
1 tablespoon of plain almonds

Shakshooka
1 whole egg, 1 egg white
30 g of goat cheese or feta cheese
1 diced tomato
¼ cup chopped chives
½ cup of chopped onion, paprika, pepper, salt

- In a pan on medium heat, stir-fry onion and chives for 2–3 minutes in 1 tablespoon of vegetable oil. Add the tomato; after two minutes, add the egg.
- Add cheese and spices at the end.

- You can have it with 1 piece brown toast or 1 whole wheat pita bread

Morning Fresh

In the blender, put ½–1 cup of Greek yogurt, 1 unpeeled cucumber, mint leaves, ½ cup of green cantaloupe, 1–2 tablespoons of protein powder (iso protein), ice cubes. Blend.

Poached Eggs with Veggies

1 cup of vegetable (pan fried or boiled): 1 small potato, 1 diced zucchini, 1 cup of diced mushroom

You add on the veggies 1–2 poached eggs with spices and fine herbs.

Cocoa Parfait

½–1 cup of Greek yogurt
½ cup of pineapple or papaya
30 g of dark chocolate chopped
1 tablespoon of plain seeds

You add the ingredients by layers.

Here are some lunch recipes.

Quiche

½ cup of chopped parsley
¼ cup of chopped dill
1 shredded carrot (medium size) raw
1 shredded zucchini, raw
1–2 eggs
1–2 tablespoons of whole wheat oat
Spices (salt and pepper)

- Grease a pan with vegetable oil.

- Mix all the ingredients, and place them in the pan to be baked for 20–30 minutes at 350°C. (You give it some time to rest before serving)

Lentil Salad
2 cups baby spinach, ½–1 cup of cooked lentil, 2–4 tablespoons of goat or feta cheese, 1 chopped tomato, ½ cup of chopped chives, 1 grilled chopped eggplant, spices, extra-virgin olive oil, and balsamic vinegar, salt and pepper.

Tuna Sandwich
1–2 pieces brown toast
tuna in water, 120–180 g (organic is better)
½ avocado
2 tablespoon of lemon
pepper
lettuce

- Mix the tuna with avocado, lemon, pepper.
- Make the sandwich with lettuce.

Mixed Veggies and Minced Meat (Chelo Fry)
1 boiled sweet potato, diced
150–250 g lean minced meat
1–2 diced tomato
½ cup chopped parsley
½ chopped onion
1–2 tablespoon of vegetable oil
paprika, pepper, salt

- In a pan, stir-fry on & medium heat onion and parsley for 3–4 minutes.
- Add tomato and minced meat for 3–5 minutes. At the end, add the sweet potato.
- Add the spices, stir for another 4–5 minutes, and serve.

Here are some dinner recipes.

1 sliced avocado
½ boiled corn
120–180 g chicken marinated in yogurt, curcuma, lemon, ginger (2–12 hours of marination) and grill it
½ cup of chopped coriander
1–2 cups of lettuce
lemon or balsamic vinegar
fine herbs

- Grill the chicken and cut it in pieces.
- Prepare the salad: lettuce with avocado, coriander, corn. Add the chicken, and add the lemon or balsamic vinegar and fine herbs.

Tes Tes with Chickpeas
1 cup of boiled chickpeas (add cumin and pepper and 1–2 tablespoons of lemon juice)
½ cup of low-fat yogurt
1 tablespoon of roasted pine nuts, chopped
½ cup of chopped parsley
1 small whole wheat pita grilled in the oven and shredded randomly
1 tablespoon of extra-virgin olive oil

- In a bowl, put in the chickpeas; add the parsley, yogurt, and pine nuts; then add the bread at the top and the olive oil.
- You can eat it by layers or mix up all the ingredients

Eggplant Salad
1 grilled eggplant (unpeeled and sliced)
½ cup of chopped parsley
2 cup baby spinach
1 diced tomato
1 chopped green pepper

30–60 g of feta cheese
½ cup of pomegranate
1 tablespoon of virgin olive oil
1 tablespoon of pomegranate sauce
1 tablespoon of balsamic vinegar
pepper

Mix all the ingredients together, add the olive oil, the pomegranate, and the balsamic vinegar

Fish Soup
1 chopped onion
2–3 chopped tomatoes
3 cloves garlic, chopped
1 tablespoon vegetable oil
2 tablespoons lemon juice
2 tablespoons dried mint
1 tablespoon dried oregano
120–180 g white fish (like dory)

- In a pan stir-fry the mint and oregano in the oil, 2–3 minutes (medium heat).
- Add onion and garlic, 3–4 minutes.
- Add tomato with pepper, 2 minutes.
- Add the fish, cover the pan, and cook it in the oven 350°C for 15–20 minutes.
- Add salt and lemon before serving.

These are some recipes to increase the metabolism. You should have one of these recipes during the day.

In the blender, add the following:
mint leaves 15–20
1 tablespoon of lemon juice
2 teaspoons of lemon zest

1 unpeeled cucumber
1 tablespoon of aloe vera gel or ¼ cup of aloe vera juice
stevia
1 cup of water or sparkling water
Ice cubes

In the blender, add the following:
½ cup of beetroot juice
2 teaspoons of fresh ginger
½ cup of carrot juice
parsley leaves
ice cubes

In the blender, add the following:
½ cup of pineapple
¼ cup of grapefruit juice
¼ cup baby spinach
1 tablespoon of aloe vera gel or ¼ cup of aloe vera juice
ice cubes

In the blender, add the following:
½ cup of apple juice
½ teaspoon of cinnamon
½ teaspoon of cloves (powder)
1 teaspoon of chia seeds
1 cup of sparkling water
ice cubes

In the blender, add the following:
½ cup of tomato juice
½ teaspoon chili powder
½ teaspoon of ginger
1–2 celery
ice cubes

In the blender, add the following:
½ cup of carrot juice
¼ grapefruit or ¼ cup of amla
leaves of coriander
stevia
ice cubes

In the blender, add the following:
½ cup karela juice
½ cup aloe vera juice or 2 tablespoon of aloe vera gel
½ cup of apple juice
1 tablespoon of lemon

- It is important to choose 100 percent fresh juice or natural 100 percent without any preservative or artificial agents.
- If you take any medicine for hypertension or high cholesterol or anything else, please don't take grapefruit; have orange instead. To be sure, ask your pharmacist or doctor.
- Karela (bitter cucumber) and amla (fruit) have bitter tastes but are rich in antioxidants and increase the metabolism.
- Kindly respect all quantities. If you like to sweeten up your juices or drinks, use stevia or honey or a bit of Canadian maple syrup.
- If you have any kidney diseases and/or water quantity should be counted during the day, please talk to your healthcare provider before doing this or any diet.
- If you take any medication that should limit your water quantity or any food items written in this book, please talk to your healthcare provider before following this diet.
- Weight loss is not magic, it takes time because our body is not a machine, lets respect it. Those diets aim to change few of your lifestyle and nutrition habits. Meanwhile, it'll help you lose the extra weight gradually.
- If you have any allergy, heartburn, digestion problems, etc. and/or intolerance to any food item mentioned in this book or

you believe, there is a possible interaction between recipes ingredients and your disease, or any vitamins or medication you take, kindly consult with your healthcare provider first.

- Quantities:
  1 tablespoon =15 ml
  1 teaspoon =5 ml
  1 cup=250 ml or 8 oz
  30g= 1 oz
  Dressing: lemon and/or lemon zest and/or balsamic vinegar
  2 tablespoons and 1-2 tablespoons of extra virgin olive oil

"AVOID" LIST

(4–5 times per month, with regular serving size)

fried food
processed food
breaded food
salty food
sugary food
bakeries
commercial cakes and cookies
food prepared with too many sauces
white flour
alcohol
commercial fruit drinks

REFERENCES

Gardner JW, Death by water intoxication. Mil Med. 2002

Speedy DB et al, Exercise associated hyponatremia: a review. Emerg Med, 2001

http://Mayoclinic.com Mayoclinic.com, Water: How mauch should you drink every day? April 2010

NPR. Org: Five myths about drinking water, Allison Aubrey, April 2008

http://ScientificAmerican.com ScientificAmerican.com, Strange but true: drinking too much water can kill, Coco Ballantyne, June 2007

Min A Joo et al, Hyponatremia cause by excessive intake of water as a form of child abuse. Annal of Ped Endo and Metab, 2013.